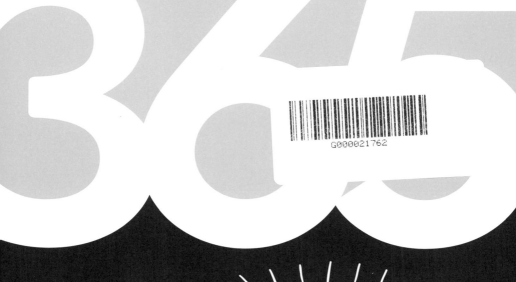

365

ways to be FITTER

365 WAYS TO BE FITTER

Copyright © Summersdale Publishers Ltd, 2019

Text by Claire Chamberlain

An Hachette UK Company
www.hachette.co.uk

Vie Books, an imprint of Summersdale Publishers Ltd
Part of Octopus Publishing Group Limited
Carmelite House
50 Victoria Embankment
LONDON
EC4Y 0DZ
UK

www.summersdale.com

Printed and bound in the Czech Republic

ISBN: 978-1-78685-758-3

Substantial discounts on bulk quantities of Summersdale books are available to corporations, professional associations and other organisations. For details contact general enquiries: telephone: +44 (0) 1243 771107 or email: enquiries@summersdale.com.

Neither the author nor the publisher can be held responsible for any loss or claim arising out of the use, or misuse, of the suggestions made herein. Consult your doctor before undertaking any new forms of exercise.

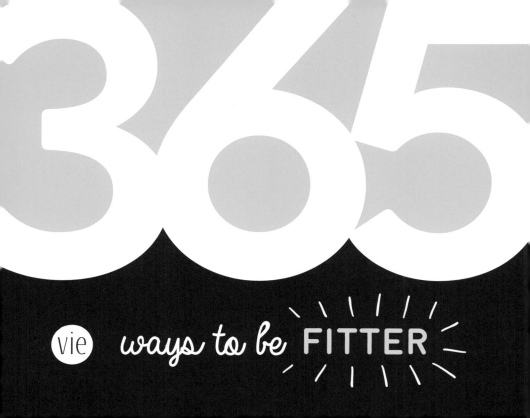

365

vie *ways to be* FITTER

1

Deciding to get fit is the first step! Now, do everything you can to make it easy for yourself to follow through with your intentions.

Think about why you want to get fitter. Is it to feel more energised? To improve your mental health? To shed some weight? Having a clearly defined reason will help you stick with it.

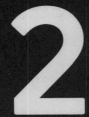

Write down your main reason for getting fitter
and pin it up somewhere you'll see it daily, such as
next to your bed or on the fridge door.

**Make exercise a habit, just like
brushing your teeth or washing your hair.**

Schedule exercise time into your diary. When it's written
down in black and white, you're more likely to prioritise it.

Set yourself a tangible goal, such as a 5K race or an 800-m swim – it's a great way to stay motivated.

Tell other people about your fitness goal – it will make you accountable and therefore more likely to achieve it.

8

Everyone who exercises regularly was once
a beginner. Start today and join the club!

That first fitness session is often the hardest because
you're entering unknown territory – so get it over with!

Remember that doing *something* is always
better than doing nothing – even five
minutes of exercise has a positive impact.

Enlist a friend to exercise with!
You'll help to spur each other on.

12

Stop telling yourself you can't do it. Wanting to get fitter is the first step towards proving that you can.

Don't compare yourself to others. This is your fitness journey, so take it at your own pace.

13

Keep a fitness journal recording the exercise you've completed and how each session makes you feel.

Celebrate each victory, however small. If two weeks ago you couldn't jog to the end of your road, but now you can, that's a big deal. Well done!

16

Embrace the sessions that feel challenging – they're helping you get fitter and stronger.

17

Remember, in order to get fitter, you must push yourself just beyond your comfort zone.

Small daily or weekly improvements are the key to long-term success. It all adds up!

Try visualisation. Imagine exercising and feeling great: what can you see, feel and hear? Visualising your workout positively will motivate you to make it a reality.

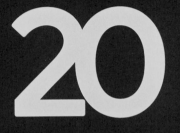

20

When looking for motivation to get fitter, come from a place of self-love, not self-loathing.

When the going gets tough, remember why you started.

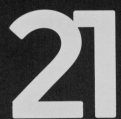

21

Prove to yourself that you can do it.

Every day is a new opportunity to
get fitter and feel stronger.

24

Lay out your workout kit before going to bed, then put it on as soon as you get up in the morning. Once it's on, you might as well make the most of it!

25

Struggling to get going? Tell yourself you'll exercise for just five minutes. Five minutes is better than nothing, and chances are you'll keep going once you've started.

26

Believe in yourself. You can do this!

27

It can be daunting starting a new
exercise regime – so be brave and
step out of that comfort zone.

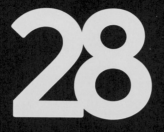

28

If you feel like skipping an exercise session, ask yourself whether you will regret it if you do.

Remember, pledging to get fitter is a fantastic way to look after your health – both mental and physical.

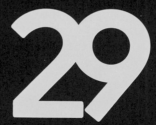

29

30

Start small. No one is expecting you to run a marathon or swim a kilometre straight away!

31

Download a beginner's training schedule in your chosen activity, such as a 0–5K running plan. Following a plan is a great way to boost your confidence and chart your progress.

32

Aim for the recommended 150 minutes of exercise per week – just five 30-minute sessions.

If you're new to exercise, or haven't worked on your fitness for a while, build up slowly to your target of 150 minutes of exercise a week.

When you first start out, aim low! Try five to ten minutes of exercise per session. Easing yourself in gently will give your body time to adapt.

35

Building fitness means different things to different people. What does it mean to you? For example, is it about building strength or being able to run 5 km?

36

Take your current fitness level into consideration. If you are pretty active already, you will likely find a new activity such as running or cycling easier. If you currently lead a mostly sedentary lifestyle, start by increasing your activity with daily brisk walks.

37

Whatever your main fitness priority, ensure
your exercise plan is well rounded, by incorporating
sessions each week that help to improve strength,
cardiovascular fitness and flexibility. You could do this
easily with a weekly yoga session, a strength session and
two cardio sessions, such as cycling or brisk walking.

38

**Keep your goal in mind – such as your ideal body
shape – but don't forget what's great about yourself right now.**

39

Remember, your body is amazing... and it's about to take you on an exciting fitness journey!

40

Don't be disheartened if you start working out but don't seem to lose weight. Muscle is denser than fat, so even though you're becoming leaner, the scales might not register the change.

41

Take monthly photos of yourself, or record some body measurements, to help track your progress.

42

Ask for guidance. If you are new to the gym, book an induction session, or if you sign up to a new fitness class, make sure the instructor knows you're a beginner.

43

Consider a session with a personal trainer – they will be able to tailor a workout programme to your current fitness level and goal.

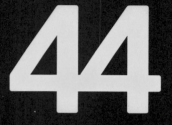

44

Don't feel intimidated! You have just as much right to be working out as anyone else.

Don't copy others. Running faster than is comfortable or lifting weights heavier than you can manage, just because other people can, will be demoralising and you could injure yourself. This is *your* journey – do it your way.

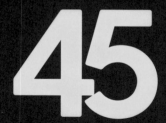

45

Relish the enthusiasm you feel in the first few weeks
of a new fitness regime. It's all new and exciting,
so sticking with it will seem like a breeze...

... but prepare for motivation to drop away in
the third or fourth week. Don't panic, it's common!
Stick with your routine until it becomes a habit.

48

Embarrassed to be sweaty, red-faced and out of breath? Don't be! This is what working out looks like. Instead, congratulate yourself on a great effort.

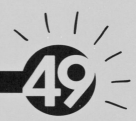

49

No one is looking at you. Trust us! Everyone else is caught up with their own workout.

50

Confused about fitness terminology? Don't be afraid to ask what something means.

51

Cardio exercise is one of the main categories of exercise and should definitely feature in any fitness regime. Any exercise that raises your heart rate, such as running or swimming, is considered cardio. You know it's a cardio workout if it leaves you breathless!

52

Strength training refers to a fitness session that works your muscles. Try to alternate workouts between cardio and strength training as much as you can.

53

Strength workouts often talk about 'reps' and 'sets'.
A rep (repetition) is one complete motion of a particular
move, such as one squat. A set is a group of reps.

54

'Resistance' refers to how much weight your body is
resisting in order to complete the workout move. For example, an 8-kg
kettle bell means you are working with 8 kg of resistance.

55

Try body-weight exercises – moves that use your
own body weight as resistance, for example, press-ups.
No weights or gym equipment are required, so no excuses!

56

'Circuits' refers to a series of different exercises performed at a high intensity for a short amount of time, with minimal rest in between. Have a look at your local gym for a good introductory class.

Try high-intensity interval training, or HIIT: a short but intense workout session, designed to get your heart rate up. It's an effective way to burn fat quickly.

57

58

Interval training can be applied to many different activities and refers to a period of work followed by a period of rest, repeated a number of times. In running, this could be three minutes of fast running, followed by two minutes of jogging or brisk walking, repeated six times.

59

Include some isometric (static) exercises – such as a plank or wall sit – in your workout for an easy way to increase the strength of certain muscles. No equipment needed!

60

Plyometric exercises refer to explosive, jumping movements, such as burpees. They are great for increasing your power and improving muscular strength while also giving your metabolism a boost.

61

RPE stands for 'rate of perceived exertion'. It's measured on a scale of one to ten. Most long workouts should be done at a level four or five, with bursts of up to seven or eight for short periods.

Choose an activity that you enjoy –
then exercise will never feel like a chore.

**A great choice of exercise for you should
feel fun, challenging and exciting.**

Your chosen activity should be something you feel
compelled to take part in or improve at.

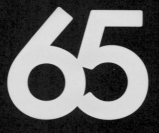

65

Remember, it pays to think outside the box when it comes to fitness!

66

If slogging it out in the gym or swimming lengths of the pool isn't your thing, why not consider something more adventurous, such as rock climbing, boxing, dancing, horse-riding or aerial skills?

If you love the idea of exercising with others, why not consider a team sport – football, hockey, netball or basketball are all accessible and popular options.

Consider your local environment – can you incorporate it into your fitness regime? If you live near the sea, perhaps water sports or wild swimming interests you. Canals are great to cycle along, parks are ideal for some off-road running, bootcamp classes or ball games, while city gyms usually offer a wide variety of classes.

69

Whatever your chosen sport or activity, it's a great idea to work on your overall strength too, so you can get the most out of it.

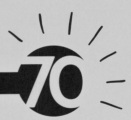

70

Working on your core, arm and leg strength will not only help you feel fitter for your chosen sport, but you'll also tone up!

71

You don't need a costly gym membership to work on your strength – do simple body-weight exercises in the comfort of your own home.

72

Here's a quick home workout you can do in your living room: run through three sets of squats, lunges, planks, press-ups and tricep dips. Start with 10 reps per set and work up to 25.

73

Do your body-weight exercises two or three times a week – in about four weeks you'll notice the improvement.

74

**Whatever activity you try, joining a club
or group can make a big difference, both
to your commitment and enjoyment.**

75

You can find official clubs or informal groups for
a whole range of activities, from running and cycling,
through to open-water swimming and hiking, so
have a look online to find one that's right for you.

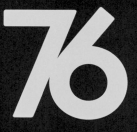

76

Training with other like-minded people is a brilliant way to boost your motivation.

If you're new to a sport, you can learn a lot from those in a club who have been doing it for years – so ask for their insider tips!

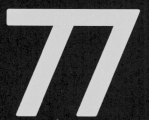

77

Make sure you choose a club or group that feels right for you – it definitely isn't one size fits all.

Email or call a club and ask questions – do they cater for beginners? Is there a social element? At what speed do they run/swim/cycle?

80

Most clubs or groups will let you attend a session or two before committing, so try before you sign up.

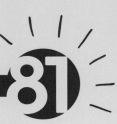

If you like the club's vibe, you've found your tribe!

82

Walking is free, convenient and one
of the simplest ways to get fitter!

83

The beauty of walking is you can do it
virtually anywhere! Whether in a city or
the countryside, home or abroad, alone,
with a group or pushing a buggy, walking
is a highly accessible fitness pursuit.

84

Walking briskly counts towards your recommended
150 minutes of exercise a week.

85

Brisk walking equates to roughly 3 miles (5 km) an hour,
but fitter people should aim for 4 miles (6.5 km) an hour.

86

Start introducing more walking into your everyday life:
for example, walk instead of driving short distances.

87

Once you're used to walking for an hour or so, why not plan some day hikes? It's a great way to add some adventure to your weekend!

If you want to boost your upper-body fitness, try Nordic walking. This involves using walking poles to harness the power of your upper body.

88

89

Hiking refers to walking along off-road trails, sometimes hilly, mountainous or coastal ones, and is a brilliant way to get back in touch with nature. It's breathtaking – in more ways than one!

90

Check out local walking groups. There are groups for everything from fitness walking to rambling, and you could even take a walking holiday.

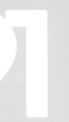

91

Have joint or mobility problems? Try walking in water! Many local swimming pools hold aqua walking or aqua aerobics classes.

Running outside for the first time can seem daunting, but don't panic. Running is empowering and energising. Simply focus on what you're doing and don't worry about anybody else.

Before you start running, ensure you're comfortable walking briskly for at least 30 minutes and make sure you have the right kit.

94

The best way to start running is to introduce several short jogs into a 30-minute walk. For example, walk for five minutes, jog for one minute and repeat five times.

Try to do your run/walk session three times a week.

96

As you get fitter, gradually increase the running intervals and decrease the walking intervals.

97

Remember, walk breaks aren't cheating! In fact, walk breaks are a great way to help you push your mental and physical barriers, meaning you can cover a greater distance. Even some top endurance runners take walk breaks.

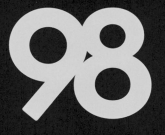

98

Even if you can currently only jog for a minute or two, you're still lapping everyone on the sofa.

Think only super-svelte people can run? Think again. Runners are an eclectic bunch, so whatever your body shape or size, you can do it.

99

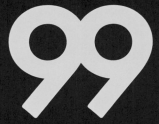

Enter a 5K or 10K race, or even a fun run,
to help you stay motivated.

Download a beginner's training plan and get stuck in!

Try parkrun – weekly, timed 5K events held at local parks
every weekend, with a sociable, inclusive vibe.

Slow down! One of the biggest mistakes new runners make is going too fast. Aim to run at 'conversational' pace – the speed at which you could still chat comfortably while running.

To improve your stamina, try a threshold session: after a warm-up jog, run at a pace that verges on uncomfortable – RPE effort level six or seven out of ten – for three to five minutes, then walk or jog to recover for several minutes. Repeat five times.

105

Hill sessions are great for building strength and fitness! After a warm-up jog, run up a hill for 45 to 60 seconds, then jog or walk back down to recover. Repeat five to ten times.

106

Bored with the treadmill or road running? Try heading off-road! Running along a trail or even through a park is great for both the mind and body.

107

Don't be intimidated by the idea of trail running. A track through a flat field or park counts – you don't have to run up a mountain!

108

For something different, try an obstacle course. This involves running a route (often around 5 km) which is dotted with a series of obstacles to tackle, often involving teamwork, silliness and a lot of mud.

109

Got race-day nerves? Take some deep breaths. Acknowledge how far you've come. And remember, if it's your first race, you are guaranteed a personal best time!

110

Remember, it doesn't matter how far or how fast you go. If you run, then you are a runner.

Yoga is a spiritual practice, which focuses on uniting the mind, body and spirit (the word 'yoga' is rooted in the Sanskrit 'yuj', meaning 'to unite'). While its essence is spiritual, yoga has become hugely popular in the West, blending physical postures ('asanas') with meditation.

Yoga can be used to help create a sense of balance within the body, improving flexibility and strength while also evoking a sense of peace, stillness and well-being.

113

There are lots of different forms of yoga, including Hatha (gentle, slow yoga); Vinyasa (matching movement to the breath, or 'flow' yoga); and Ashtanga (more physically demanding).

114

Anyone can start practising yoga, regardless of their current strength or flexibility level. New to yoga? Search for a Hatha, relaxation or beginner class.

TIP 5

There are so many health benefits to practising yoga. These include increased flexibility, strength and balance, improved digestion, a strengthened immune system and better sleep. What's not to love?

TIP 6

Yoga is wonderful at helping you to overcome negative or self-limiting beliefs: you are not too inflexible, too old or too overweight. Yoga is for everyone!

TIP 7

In yoga, as in any activity, don't push yourself beyond your current physical limitations. Improvement will come with time, practice and patience.

118

If you're new to yoga, it is best to work with a qualified instructor first to avoid performing exercises incorrectly.

119

Once you've got the hang of the basic positions, try developing a 10-minute routine you can perform to either prepare you for the day, or to relax you before bed.

120

Learn a variation of the Sun Salutation so that you can practise whenever you have some spare time – it can be as quick and gentle as you like, and can be fitted into five minutes.

121

Swimming is a fun and low-impact sport -- and it can also provide an intense full-body workout!

Can't swim? It's never too late to learn! Book some adult beginner lessons, and learn alongside others in your position.

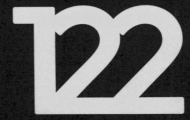

122

123

Even if you can swim, consider investing in a few lessons to help build your confidence and improve your technique in a variety of strokes.

124

When you first start, focus on the stroke that feels most natural to you, to help build your confidence. Stay calm while in the water. The more relaxed you are, the more natural your strokes will feel.

125

Steady, controlled breathing is a crucial element of confident swimming. Practise submerging your face and exhaling fully underwater several times before you begin.

126

Your body position in the water plays a big part in how effortless swimming will feel for you. Aim to stay flat, with your whole body on top of the water, rather than letting your feet and hips sink down, which creates more resistance.

127

If you're a competent swimmer,
don't confine yourself to lengths of the pool!
Why not give open-water swimming a go?

128

If swimming in open water, such as the sea or
a lake, always do so with a friend, as wild swimming
alone can be dangerous. Make sure you're swimming in
a safe place where there are no currents or rip tides.

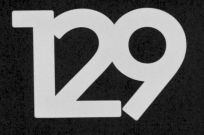

129

Remember, there are no lanes in the open water! Practise 'sighting', by finding an object in the distance to focus on and heading for that, so you remain on course.

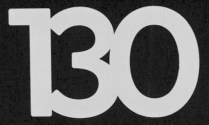

130

Sign up for a triathlon to encourage you to develop your running, cycling and swimming for an all-round fitness boost.

131

Cycling is a great way to get fit while also enabling
you to cover greater distances than running
or hiking. Perfect for an adventure!

132

Before you get started, make sure your bike is in peak
condition and set up to suit your body – an expert at a
cycling shop will be able to help you. At the very least,
ensure your tyres are fully pumped up (it takes much
more effort cycling on under-inflated tyres!).

133

Never cycle while listening to music, as you need to be fully aware of the environment around you, and stay safe by wearing a helmet and high-visibility clothing.

134

Take every opportunity to cycle whenever you can – even just a five-minute trip to the shops instead of walking will improve your stamina and strength.

135

If you love cycling but your commute is too long to switch it for a bike ride, why not invest in a folding bike so you can get off the train or bus a few stops early and cycle the rest of the way?

136

If you're heading out for long-distance rides, it's a good idea to learn the basics in bike maintenance, such as removing a wheel, repairing a puncture or oiling a chain. Sign up to a maintenance course or educate yourself with online tutorials.

137

Learn how to use your gears correctly for more effortless cycling. As a general rule, when climbing a hill, shift into a lower gear; when descending, use a higher gear.

138

Fancy an adventure? Try heading off-road to boost your fitness further and embrace the mud! It's a great way to explore.

139

If you fancy a more technical off-road challenge, give single-track mountain biking a go. This is along a track roughly the width of the bike and often includes hills, tree roots and rocks to navigate for extra excitement.

140

Climb a mountain! You will be motivated to get more active as you prepare for the challenge, and the actual act itself will be one big all-round workout, with an epic view at the end.

141

There are so many different sporting and fitness options out there, you are bound to find the perfect fit for you. If one doesn't work for you, don't worry, there are plenty of other things to try!

142

Fancy an indoor workout? While you could hit the gym, other more interesting options include boxing, kick-boxing, ballroom dancing or bouldering at a climbing centre.

143

For adrenaline seekers, why not look to see if there are any watersports clubs or centres nearby where you could try surfing, wakeboarding, windsurfing, rafting or canyoning – sports so fun you'll forget you're exercising!

144

If you like the idea of spending time on the water rather than in it, you could try kayaking, stand-up paddle boarding (SUP) or even sailing.

145

Love the idea of cycling, but prefer an indoor environment? Try a spinning class – a group class set to music where you sit on stationary bikes that use resistance to create a heart-racing workout.

146

Horse-riding is a wonderful option for animal lovers with a head for heights!

Bootcamp classes are becoming increasingly popular – they offer a gym-style workout in the great outdoors, complete with plenty of mud!

147

148

If you want to combine fitness with learning a new skill (one that will be a great talking point!), search for your nearest circus or aerial skills class.

149

New parent? Check out classes that allow you to bring baby along! Options include BuggyFit, where you exercise outdoors with your baby in the buggy, and dance or Zumba classes where you dance with your baby in a sling.

150

Spend five minutes stretching or performing some gentle exercises as soon as you get out of bed.

151

Perform squats, lunges or wall press-ups in the kitchen while waiting for the kettle to boil or the microwave to ding. How many can you complete?

152

To improve your balance, try standing on one leg while performing daily tasks, such as brushing your teeth or peeling vegetables. Remember to swap legs! Good balance is vital for stability and injury prevention when exercising.

153

Make TV time more active! Instead of lounging on the sofa in front of your favourite box set, perform a strength and conditioning session while you watch, or see if you can hold a plank for the duration of the ad break.

154

Stair-climbing is great for raising your heart rate and toning your bum! So make the most of your stairs. Jog up them every time you use them, if you can do so safely, or see how many times you can walk up and down them in five minutes.

155

Invest in a workout DVD or search online for short home workouts – great for an evening in, or if you're nervous about joining a gym.

156

Got a spare five minutes? Switch on that radio and dance! Dancing to upbeat music is not only good for your body, but it will put a smile on your face, too.

157

Heading to the local shops? Walk there and then carry your shopping bags home instead of driving – a great (and practical) way to build strength.

158

Instead of asking someone else to grab your jumper from upstairs or a drink from the kitchen, get them yourself! Movement is better than staying sedentary and every little helps.

159

Housework counts towards your daily activity, as long as it builds up a sweat (think scrubbing the bathtub vigorously rather than standing still doing the washing up!).

Gardening is physically intensive and a great all-round
workout that doesn't feel like traditional 'exercise'
– so get out those secateurs!

Your daily commute is a great opportunity to exercise!
If your commute is less than three miles, walking briskly
to and from work every day is a good option.

If you have a long commute, consider getting off the
bus a few stops earlier, or parking further away from the
office, so you can spend more time on your feet.

163

When walking, make sure your pace is brisk so it counts as aerobic exercise.

164

Consider running all or part of the way home from work (or to work, if you have access to showers or won't arrive all sweaty!). Run-commuting is a brilliant workout and a great way to fit a more strenuous cardio session into your day.

165

Whether running, walking or cycling, plan your commute in advance on a map – you don't want to get lost and turn up late.

166

Walking or running to work is a great way to find new routes – you might find yourself in parks, green spaces or even alongside rivers or canals.

When commuting by train or bus, try standing for all or some of your journey (this might be necessary anyway!). Use your core strength to keep yourself stable while on the move.

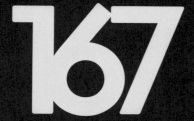

167

168

Place a stepper or pedal exerciser underneath your desk, so you can keep moving your legs while sitting.

169

Take the stairs rather than an escalator or, if there's no alternative, walk up the escalator rather than letting it do all the work.

170

Avoid using lifts if possible. Taking the stairs will not only help you tone up, but will increase your heart rate too – great for boosting your cardiovascular fitness!

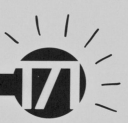

While sitting at your desk, set an hourly alert on your phone or computer to remind you to get up and take a brief walk.

172

Replace your usual office chair with a stability ball – great for improving core strength and balance while you work.

173

Take every opportunity to move more during your working day: offer to do the tea round or walk the longer route to the photocopier.

T74

Make the most of your
lunch break by heading out
for a brisk walk or run.

T75

Is there a gym near your office? Why
not enrol in a lunchtime fitness class?
There's nothing like a spinning session
to wake you up for the afternoon!

T76

Stretching is not only great for flexibility,
but it helps to relieve stress and tension
too – perfect for the office! Take some time
to stretch regularly throughout the day.

Why not suggest a 'walk and talk' meeting
instead of a sedentary one?

Organise a sponsored fitness challenge with
colleagues, such as a charity 5K or bike ride –
great for team building and motivation!

Suggest a game of rounders in the local park at lunchtime
or after work – it could quickly become a regular event.

180

It's wonderful to involve your loved ones when you make the decision to get fitter – that way you can help boost the health of your whole family or circle of friends!

181

Suggest that your partner or friend join you in your new fitness pursuit – go for a hike, bike ride or jog together.

182

If your exercise partner isn't keen on your chosen activity, why not mix and match? You could run while they cycle alongside you for encouragement.

183

Try a circuits routine with a partner! One of you runs a lap of the park while the other performs a set of lunges. Then swap. Repeat with squats, planks, press-ups and sit-ups.

184

There are lots of ways to involve kids in your fitness quest – especially during your usual day-to-day routines. For example:

185

Always walk them to school instead of driving or taking the bus.

186

Take your kids out on their scooters or bikes more often during the week – you can walk briskly, jog or cycle along with them.

187

Get involved in trips to the playground! Pushing your kids on the swings, hanging from the monkey bars with them, and playing games of chase, catch or frisbee all count towards your daily activity.

188

If your children are young, show them how to use a skipping rope, or if they're older, try skipping rope competitions.

189

By getting active yourself, you'll become a fantastic role model for your family – so keep it up!

190

There are so many physical and mental benefits of exercise, you will soon feel inspired to stick with it to improve your health. It just takes the first few weeks of perseverance before you'll feel the addictive benefits!

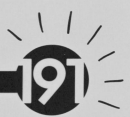

191

Alongside physical activity, eating a healthy, balanced diet is an important part of maintaining a healthy weight.

192

Remember: exercising regularly will leave
you with more energy, not less!

193

The number of calories you burn depends
on your chosen activity, intensity level and weight.
But as an example, the average person will burn
80–160 calories for every mile they walk.

194

Instead of meeting a friend for dinner or a drink, suggest going for a walk together – or even shopping, which is great for you physically (though maybe not financially).

195

According to the World Health Organization, people who do regular physical activity have lower rates of all-cause mortality, coronary heart disease, stroke, type 2 diabetes, metabolic syndrome, colon and breast cancer, and depression.

196

Regular exercise improves your cardiorespiratory and muscular fitness.

197

Keeping active through regular exercise has been shown to lower blood pressure as much as some blood pressure medications.

198

Regular exercise is a great way to lower your cholesterol, helping to ward off potential heart disease.

199

Regular high-impact, weight-bearing activity, such as running, helps to strengthen your bones, reducing your risk of developing osteoporosis. Regular exercise will also cut your risk of a hip or vertebral fracture.

200

Even a small amount of cardiovascular exercise, such as light jogging for ten minutes a day, could increase your life expectancy by up to six years!

Want to stay injury-free in later life? Then keep exercising!
Good physical fitness in older adults improves stability,
reducing the chance of falls by 30 per cent.

Regular exercise can result in more radiant, healthy-
looking skin, due to improved blood circulation and
sweat expelling oil or dirt trapped in your pores.

Activities that improve flexibility and core strength,
such as Pilates or yoga, will help to improve your posture.

204

Exercise has been shown to relieve chronic pain, as well as increasing pain tolerance and decreasing pain perception. It has also been proven to reduce the intensity of period pain in women. Try a brisk walk or gentle jog to ease symptoms.

205

Regular moderate exercise could help to boost your immune system, so get active to ward off that pesky cold!

206

Exercise helps you to drop off to sleep more easily and can also improve your sleep patterns.

207

Frequent activity can boost your brainpower! Exercise helps to pump more oxygen-rich blood to the hippocampus – the area of the brain responsible for learning.

208

Regular aerobic exercise is one of the best ways to reduce your risk of developing dementia, according to scientists.

209

Even just ten minutes of brisk walking can improve positivity, alertness and energy levels.

210

It's a fact that physical activity can make you happier! Exercise stimulates the brain into producing endorphins (the 'happy' hormone), boosting a sense of mental well-being. Many doctors now prescribe exercise as a way of treating mild to moderate depression – so if you're feeling low, get active!

211

Invite friends to the park for a picnic and games day, rather than sitting still inside. Or swap a cinema date for a beach walk.

212

Add some small dumbbells or kettlebells (or improvise with weighty objects) to your workout for an extra shot of strength training.

213

The combination of exercise and the natural world has been shown to be the best way to improve mental well-being, so try exercising outdoors in nature – known as 'green exercise'.

214

Following an exercise plan and getting fitter gives you an enormous sense of achievement. It will boost your self-esteem and your confidence levels and is a great stress-buster.

215

Exercise helps you recognise your own strength and resilience, so you're better able to cope with challenges in other areas of your life.

216

Exercise is a great way to boost your social life – joining an exercise class, club, group or team could see you making a whole new set of friends!

217

Exercise has been shown to increase your sex drive – great for strengthening your relationship with your partner.

218

If you're in need of some fresh ideas for a particular project or problem, get active. Physical exercise boosts creativity!

219

Exercise can help you live in the moment. As you work out, focus on your breathing, your immediate surroundings and the activity you're doing – this will help you become more mindful.

220

Going for a walk after dinner will help you to digest the meal, give you some downtime every day and build up your daily step count.

221

Whenever you take a phone call, go for a walk or perform some stretches or gentle exercises at the same time.

222

Walk the dog! Or, if you don't have one, ask if friends or neighbours would appreciate you helping out with theirs. It's a stressbuster and will give your walk more purpose and energy.

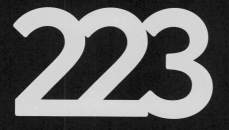

223

When food shopping, take a basket rather than a trolley – your arms will appreciate the extra workout.

Fuelling your body correctly both before and after exercise is a vital component when it comes to improving your fitness. Eating the correct foods will ensure you see the best results.

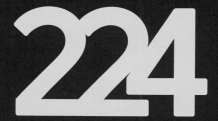

224

225

Think about your fitness goals. Do you want to tone up, build muscle, boost your energy or train for an endurance event? Each of these has different nutritional requirements, but they all require a healthy diet.

226

You're unique! That means the amount you need to eat to fuel your exercise and recovery will be unique to you, too.

227

The amount you need to eat daily will depend on several factors, including your current weight, your general daily activity level and the amount and type of exercise you're doing.

On average, guidelines suggest men should eat 2,500 calories a day. For women it's 2,000.

229

If you consume more calories than you're burning, you'll start putting on weight and this could negatively affect your fitness training.

230

If you consume significantly fewer calories than you're burning, you may feel lethargic, tired and light-headed while training, which can be dangerous.

231

Complex carbohydrates such as whole grains, legumes and starchy vegetables should form the basis of your diet, making up a third of your daily food intake.

232

Your body turns carbohydrates into glycogen, which is then stored in your muscles as fuel for exercise.

233

Try eating a combination of slow- and fast-releasing carbohydrates prior to exercise. This will give your body immediate fuel to burn, as well as stocking up your glycogen stores for later use.

234

Good pre-exercise food options include porridge topped with honey; two slices of toast with jam; cereal with milk; a banana; or a baked sweet potato with veg.

235

Some people swear by caffeine before a workout to boost energy, but it can play havoc with your stomach. It's a case of trial and error to see if it works for you.

236

Make sure you eat roughly two hours before you exercise. This will give your body enough time to digest your food properly.

If you will be working out for longer than an hour, it's a good idea to take in fuel during exercise, to keep your energy levels topped up.

237

238 Many people take energy gels, which provide a concentrated hit of fast-release carbohydrate, to fuel activities such as running or cycling.

239 Energy gels can be very sickly – if you want to give them a go, try a few different brands until you discover the most palatable for you.

240 You can fuel your exercise with ordinary foods, too. Lots of runners opt for jelly sweets, but for a healthier alternative you could go for dates or dried fruits.

241

For lower-impact activities, such as a day's hiking,
try fuelling with regular foods, such as bananas
– and a nutritious picnic, of course!

242

It's vital to keep your body well hydrated,
not only to support your fitness goals,
but for your general health and well-being.

243

The European Food Safety Authority guidelines recommend water intake of 2.5 litres daily for men, and 2 litres daily for women. Your water intake can come from both fluids and foods.

244

It's a good idea to drink water during exercise – invest in a reusable sports bottle.

245

As a general rule, it's best to drink according to thirst while exercising, so take sips of water every time you feel the need.

246

The easiest way to check whether you are adequately hydrated is to check the colour of your urine. It should be a pale straw colour.

247

It can take time for your body to absorb the fluid you drink, so aim to drink roughly 500 ml of water 3–4 hours before you exercise.

248

Top up your hydration levels half an hour before you exercise, with about 250 ml of water.

249

The amount of water you lose during exercise will be dependent on your fitness level, your exertion and the weather conditions.

250

You can lose 1–2 litres of water from your body during exercise, through sweat and expiration (breathing out), so it's important to keep your fluid levels topped up.

251

If you're exercising for more than an hour, try a sports drink – this will also replace the electrolytes (salts) lost from your body through sweat.

252

Start replacing lost fluid by drinking
a glass of water straight after exercise
to kick-start your recovery.

253

The foods you eat after an exercise session can help
your body recover, so it's important to refuel correctly.

Always aim to eat something
within 30 minutes of exercise.

It's vital to take on a higher percentage
of protein after exercise, as this is best to
repair and replenish your muscles.

The best recovery food options are reported to have
a 4:1 ratio of protein to carbohydrates.

257

Great sources of protein are lean meat, fish, seafood, eggs, beans, pulses, nuts and tofu.

258

Good post-workout food choices include peanut butter on wholegrain toast; a banana and a glass of milk; Greek yogurt topped with berries; bean chilli with rice; salmon and new potatoes; or a tofu and vegetable stir-fry with noodles.

259

Surprisingly, a glass of chocolate milk has been shown to be just as beneficial after a workout as a branded sports drink, and has the bonus of added healthy fats, carbs, protein and calcium.

It has been suggested that drinking cherry juice after a workout can reduce muscle soreness and help restore your strength quickly – plus all those antioxidants help keep you in peak physical form.

260

261

Always make sure you're taking on an adequate supply of vitamins and minerals to help support your body as you get fitter.

262

To easily boost your vitamin and mineral intake, increase the amount of fruit and veg you eat, as well as healthy fats, such as avocados and nuts. Aim to eat five to ten portions of fruit and veg daily.

263

Cardio exercise, such as running, can deplete your body's iron stores, so make sure you're getting enough. Eat plenty of beans, nuts, dried fruit, whole grains and red meat to top up your supply.

264

Vitamin D is vital to support bone health, but it's hard to get from food – your body needs sunlight to make it. Consider a year-round daily supplement to ensure you're getting enough.

265

Pick up hobbies that involve physical activity, even if they're not traditional exercise: an amateur dramatics society or crafting class such as woodworking or pottery will keep you active even when you're in 'relaxation' mode.

266

It's a good idea to invest in specialist fitness kit – it will keep you comfortable and secure as you exercise.

267

Instead of trapping sweat next to the skin, technical workout clothing wicks moisture to the outside of the fabric where it can evaporate, which keeps you dry and minimises chafing.

268

Your basic fitness wardrobe could include a technical T-shirt, lightweight waterproof jacket, running shorts, a long-sleeve base layer for cold weather and, for women, a high-impact sports bra.

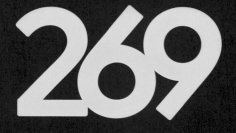

269

As a general rule, women should replace sports bras every six months.

Always look after your sports kit according to the manufacturer's instructions, to ensure it lasts well and retains its technical, sweat-wicking properties.

270

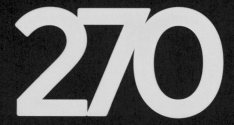

271

For exercise such as running, it's important to wear properly fitting running shoes. A specialist running shop will be able to advise you on the best shoes for your running style and gait.

272

When investing in running shoes, buy a pair that's half to a full size larger than your regular shoe size. Your feet will get warmer and swell as you run, so the extra room will prevent your toes getting squashed!

273

Your running shoes will wear out over time and their shock absorbency will decrease. It's best to replace them after 400–500 miles of use to help prevent injury.

274

An exercise belt provides a safe place for your key
(and other essentials you want with you, like a phone or
credit card) during a workout, rather than having to hold
them awkwardly or risk leaving them in the gym!

275

Want to exercise but stuck for childcare? Invest in a running
buggy! They're a great option for parents of young children
and are suitable for babies from six months of age.

276

If you're planning to exercise in the comfort of your own home, investing in some basic kit may inspire you to stick with it, and will also make your home workouts easier and more convenient.

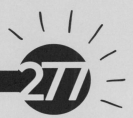

277

A yoga mat is a great purchase for all home workouts, as the non-slip surface will help keep you stable and safe.

278

Remember, you don't need to fork out lots of cash for expensive equipment – household objects or furniture can be incorporated into workouts, too.

279

Try doing triceps dips using a sturdy chair and push-ups against the wall.

280

Bottles of water or tins of baked beans make great weights!

281

Music is a great motivator.
Create a personalised workout playlist
of all your favourite upbeat tunes.

282

Wireless headphones are a great
investment if you want to exercise to music, and
you can even get Bluetooth swimming headphones
so you can listen while you're in the pool.

283

If you'll be exercising outside in low light or after dark, high-visibility kit is essential to keep you safe – try a high-vis jacket or armband. These often incorporate reflective elements, too.

284

If you're planning to invest in an expensive piece of equipment, such as a bike, do your research to make sure it's the right one for you.

285

A hybrid bike is a great beginner option if you'll mainly be cycling on roads. If you'll be mostly cycling on tracks or off-road, opt for a mountain bike.

286

Specialist cycling kit will keep you comfortable as you ride. A cycling jersey has easy-access pockets for snacks and a phone.

Always invest in a good cycling helmet to keep you safe.

287

288

You might find you prefer cycling bib shorts or tights (held up with integral braces) rather than those with an elasticated waistband, for comfort.

289

Padded cycling shorts will provide added comfort as you ride. These are essential for long journeys and spinning classes!

290

Cycling gloves are also a great idea while bike riding, to offer your hands some protection and improve your grip on the handlebars.

291

Choose holidays that involve active pursuits, such as swimming, walking or adventure sports, rather than lying on a beach. At the very least, book somewhere with a gym so you can get in a couple of workouts on your holiday to keep up your fitness regime.

292

A fitness tracker or sports watch can be great motivation, helping you stick to your exercise plan and increase your daily activity.

Did you know, you can use your phone to help you get fitter? There are a multitude of exercise apps you can download to help you on your way to achieving your fitness goal.

293

294

A swimsuit and goggles are the essentials for swimming, but there are other items that could make your swim more pleasant, such as a swimming hat, nose clip and earplugs.

295

If you're planning to swim in open water, you could invest in a wetsuit, to aid warmth, buoyancy and protection from debris.

296

In open-water swimming events or triathlons, wetsuits are mandatory if the water temperature is below 14°C. You don't always have to fork out lots of money though – many events offer the option of hiring one.

297

A sports cap is a great idea when exercising outdoors to protect your head from the sun and shade your eyes.

298

Sports-specific sunglasses are a great idea if you're exercising outdoors during spring and summer months. They are designed to stay securely in place and will help protect your eyes from harmful UV rays.

299

Sports kit can be expensive, but there's no need to go for overpriced branded items just because they look good. As long as the item has the qualities you need (if in doubt, ask a professional!) and it feels comfortable, it doesn't matter how much it costs.

300

Activities such as running can sometimes cause your clothing to chafe, especially if you plan on working out for long periods of time. Applying petroleum jelly to at-risk areas can help.

301

If you haven't exercised for a while, it's a good idea to book a physical check-up with your health professional before getting started.

302

Build up any exercise you do gradually, to give both your muscles and cardiovascular system time to adapt.

303

For running and other cardio exercise, follow the ten per cent rule: build up your weekly mileage by no more than ten per cent each week.

304

For strength and resistance work, start with just a few sets of six to eight repetitions and slowly increase either the weight you lift or the number of reps – not both simultaneously.

305

Before exercise, it's important to warm up properly to avoid injuries such as muscle tears.

306

To warm up, walk briskly or jog very gently for five minutes before performing a set of dynamic stretches.

307

Dynamic stretches are 'moving stretches', such as lunges, which help prepare the body to work out by increasing blood flow to the muscles and lubricating joints. Make sure your dynamic stretches are controlled.

308

A great set of pre-workout dynamic stretches would be walking lunges, jogging on the spot with high knees, butt kicks (jogging on the spot with your heels coming up to your bum), leg swings (forwards and back, and side to side), ankle rotations, shoulder rotations and arm rotations.

309

Never stretch cold muscles – only perform stretches after you've warmed up with a short walk or jog first.

310

Correct nutrition will help to stop you feeling faint during exercise.

311

If you suffer a mild sprain or muscle strain while exercising, try the **PRICE** principles of self-treatment at home for 48–72 hours:

312

Protection – protect the injured area from further harm, for example by using a support bandage.

313

Rest – refrain from further exercise and if possible rest the injured area.

Ice – apply an ice pack (a bag of frozen peas works well!) to the area for 10–15 minutes every few hours. Avoid ice burns by wrapping the ice pack in a tea towel first.

Compression – compression bandages will help to reduce swelling.

Elevation – as much as possible, try to keep the affected area raised above the level of your heart.

317

Never ignore persistent pain or sharp pain. If you continue to exercise through pain, it could lead to greater problems, such as a stress fracture.

318

While exercising, listen to your body. If you feel any sharp pains or if something doesn't feel right, stop.

319

If injury symptoms don't ease within 48–72 hours of applying the principles of PRICE, visit a health professional.

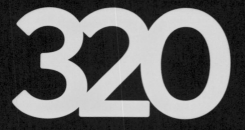

320

It's fine to exercise if you have a light cold and symptoms are above your neck (for example, a runny nose).

321

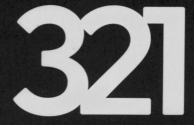

If you're unwell and symptoms are below the neck (such as a cough or chest infection), if you have a high temperature or if you're simply not feeling well enough to exercise, rest until you're better.

322

Ensure you have at least two rest days a week, to help your body recover and adapt to your new fitness routine.

323

Wear the right sports shoes! Shoes that don't offer the correct support for your gait, especially when running, can lead to muscular imbalances and shin pain. Visit a specialist sports shop, where they will be able to advise you on the correct pair for whatever activities you're undertaking.

324

Following exercise, especially after vigorous cardio such as running, it's important to cool down by walking for five minutes. This will help to prevent blood from pooling in your legs, which can make you feel faint.

325

After cooling down, perform a series of static stretches to help stop your muscles feeling tight the next day. Static stretches should be held for at least 30 seconds to a minute.

326

Stretch your quads (front thighs), hamstrings (rear thighs), calves, glutes (bum muscles) and triceps (rear arms). Unsure how to perform these? Search for an online tutorial.

327

A massage therapist can help to relax and lengthen muscles, improve blood flow and release any knots.

328

Aim to book a sports or deep-tissue massage once a month. Your body will thank you!

329

Learn to differentiate between an actual injury and the normal aches associated with exercise.

330

It's normal to feel a bit sore and stiff 24–72 hours after exercise, especially if you're not used to it! This is called delayed onset muscle soreness (DOMS).

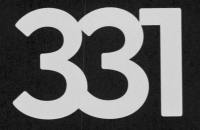

331

DOMS is nothing to worry about. In fact, it's a sign you're getting stronger and fitter: the soreness you feel is caused by micro trauma to the muscles, but your muscles then rebuild themselves stronger than before. Clever!

It's fine to exercise when you have DOMS. In fact, gentle exercise, such as a walk or swim, can help relieve it.

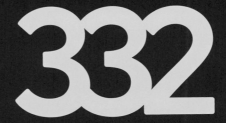

332

333

You can ease the pain of DOMS by massaging the affected area with the help of a foam roller – a large foam cylinder that can help to soothe tight muscles and sore areas.

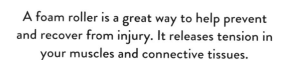

334

A foam roller is a great way to help prevent and recover from injury. It releases tension in your muscles and connective tissues.

335

To use a foam roller, simply place it on the floor and roll the affected muscles slowly over it. Never roll over joints. Search for an online tutorial for guidance.

336

Sore muscles can be relieved after exercise with a warm magnesium bath. Magnesium is a mineral that's vital for healthy muscles and it's best absorbed through the skin. Add two cups of magnesium flakes to a bath and soak for 20 minutes. Bliss!

337

Some athletes swear by ice baths to help reduce DOMS, but it doesn't have to be that severe! Simply run cold shower water over your legs for a few minutes, followed by warm water. Repeat several times.

338

Don't neglect your feet! Always keep your toenails short, trimming them straight across using nail clippers.

339

Release tension in your feet after exercise (especially after walking or running) by rolling your feet over a tennis ball or frozen water bottle.

340

Wear properly fitting sports shoes and sports socks to decrease your chance of getting blisters. If you do get a blister, remember that most blisters heal naturally within three to seven days.

341

Avoid bursting a blister, as this could lead to infection or slow the healing process.

342

If your blister bursts, let the fluid drain away, leave the skin intact and cover with a sterile dressing to help reduce the risk of infection.

343

If you're exercising outdoors in warmer months, sun damage is a real risk – don't forget to apply a high-factor sun cream.

344

Suffering with chafing clothing? Wash the affected area
with lukewarm water and antibacterial soap, and gently
pat dry before applying fragrance-free moisturiser.

345

Take good care of your sports kit and it will take care of you!
Wash everything carefully after every workout to keep it fresh.

346

It can take on average 66 days to form a new habit – so stick with it for more than two months, until your exercise routine becomes automatic.

347

Getting fitter requires dedication – remember how much you want this.

348

Struggling to keep going during a workout?
Set yourself mini goals, such as running
to the next lamppost, swimming just
one more length or keeping on pedalling
until you reach the top of the hill.

349

Try listening to an audiobook while you're
in the gym or out running. That way, you have to
keep exercising to find out what happens next!

350

In need of an extra incentive? Enter a race or fitness event and work towards earning that shiny medal.

Use your race to fundraise for a charity close to your heart. Knowing you're raising funds for an important cause is one of the best ways to keep going when you feel like quitting.

351

352

Bribe yourself to stick with it by allowing
yourself regular rewards!

353

Don't use unhealthy food as a reward. Pick things that
will enhance, not hinder, your fitness journey, such as a
massage, some new fitness kit, or clothes in your goal size.

354

If you're really not enjoying your exercise routine, or you've lost interest in it, it might be time to choose a new activity. As the saying goes, a change is as good as a rest!

355

Even if you love your exercise routine, mix it up a bit to add interest. Adding a swim, bike ride, hike or Pilates session to your week will be great for your mind and body.

356

Find a mentor in your chosen sport or activity. If possible, ask them how they motivate themselves to keep going, or read about how they have made it to the top of their game.

357

Be flexible. Everyone misses a session now and then, or has a week when they just don't feel like exercising. After all, life gets in the way sometimes! Allow yourself some leeway now and then.

358

Missing the odd session doesn't mean you've failed. It means you're human. Don't dwell on it. Just pick up where you left off and keep going.

If your fitness routine is starting to feel too easy, it's time to challenge yourself more by starting to push yourself harder.

359

Choose a mantra that will help you get through a tough session. A mantra should be short, succinct and easy to repeat in your head, to help you through. Something like: 'I am strong', or 'Fitter, stronger, healthier'.

Listen to music! There's nothing like an upbeat playlist to keep you going when you feel like quitting.

362

Whether you're at the gym, at the pool or in a class, make it your goal to be the person putting in the most effort.

363

Reframe the notion of 'discomfort' while working out. Instead of telling yourself 'This is hard', tell yourself 'This is making me stronger'.